Weight loss diet

A Comprehensive Guide to Sustainable Weight Loss and Vibrant Health

Dr. Mirabel Rosman

Introduction

Once upon a time, in a bustling city nestled between towering skyscrapers and bustling streets, there lived a young woman named Lily. Lily had always been vivacious and full of life, but as the years passed, she found herself burdened by an extra weight that seemed to weigh her down both physically and emotionally.

Despite her best efforts to shed the excess pounds, Lily found herself trapped in a cycle of fad diets, restrictive eating, and yo-yo weight fluctuations. Each attempt at weight loss left her feeling frustrated, defeated, and overwhelmed by the daunting task ahead.

One day, while scrolling through social media in search of inspiration, Lily stumbled upon a captivating story of transformation. It was the tale of Sarah, a woman who had embarked on a journey of self-discovery and weight loss, ultimately finding freedom and fulfillment through a balanced approach to nutrition and wellness.

Intrigued by Sarah's story, Lily delved deeper into the world of weight loss diets, seeking guidance and knowledge from reputable sources and experts in the field. She soon discovered that sustainable weight loss was not about deprivation or extreme measures but rather a holistic approach that prioritized nourishing the body, fostering healthy habits, and cultivating self-love and acceptance.

With newfound determination and a sense of purpose, Lily embarked on her own journey towards better health and well-being. She bid farewell to crash diets and quick fixes, instead embracing a balanced approach to nutrition that celebrated whole, nutrient-dense foods while allowing for flexibility and enjoyment.

Armed with knowledge and armed with the support of friends and loved ones, Lily began to make small, sustainable changes to her diet and lifestyle. She swapped processed snacks for fresh fruits and vegetables, traded sugary beverages for water and herbal tea, and incorporated regular exercise into her daily routine.

As the weeks and months passed, Lily's efforts began to bear fruit. She noticed her energy levels soaring, her mood lifting, and her clothes fitting more comfortably. But perhaps most importantly, she discovered a newfound sense of empowerment and self-confidence that transcended the numbers on the scale.

Through dedication, perseverance, and a willingness to embrace change, Lily embarked on a transformative journey of self-discovery and weight loss. Along the way, she learned valuable lessons about the power of nourishing the body, nurturing the mind, and honoring the journey, one step at a time.

And so, as the sun set over the city skyline, casting a warm glow over the bustling streets below, Lily stood tall and proud, knowing that she had embarked on a journey of transformation that would change her life forever.

Understanding weight loss

Understanding weight loss involves grasping the fundamental principles that govern the process of shedding excess body weight. Here are key points to consider:

1. Calories In vs. Calories Out: Weight loss occurs when you consume fewer calories than your body expends. This creates a calorie deficit, prompting your body to burn stored fat for energy.

2. Energy Balance: Energy balance is the relationship between the calories you consume (through food and beverages) and the calories you expend (through metabolism and physical activity). A negative energy balance, achieved by consuming fewer calories than you burn, leads to weight loss.

3. Metabolism: Your metabolism is the process by which your body converts food into energy. Factors such as age, gender, genetics, body composition, and activity level influence your metabolic rate, which in turn affects how many calories you burn at rest and during physical activity.

4. Nutrition: The quality and quantity of the food you eat play a significant role in weight loss. Consuming nutrient-dense foods that

are rich in fiber, protein, and healthy fats can help you feel full and satisfied while supporting overall health.

5. Physical Activity: Exercise and physical activity contribute to weight loss by increasing calorie expenditure, improving metabolic health, and preserving lean muscle mass. Incorporating both aerobic exercise and strength training into your routine can enhance weight loss efforts.

6. Behavioral Factors: Your behaviors, habits, and mindset around food and physical activity can impact your ability to lose weight. Strategies such as mindful eating, portion control, stress management, and setting realistic goals can support long-term success.

7. Sustainability: Sustainable weight loss involves making gradual, lasting changes to your diet and lifestyle that you can maintain over time. Fad diets and extreme approaches often result in temporary weight loss followed by regain, whereas sustainable habits lead to lasting results.

By understanding these principles of weight loss, you can make informed choices and develop strategies that support your journey to achieving and maintaining a healthy weight. It's essential to approach weight loss with patience, consistency, and a focus on overall health and well-being.

Weight loss diet

A weight loss diet refers to a structured eating plan designed to help individuals lose weight by reducing calorie intake and promoting fat loss while maintaining overall health and nutrition. These diets typically involve controlling portion sizes, choosing nutrient-dense foods, limiting high-calorie and processed foods, and often incorporating regular physical activity to create a calorie deficit and facilitate weight loss. The goal of a weight loss diet is to achieve sustainable and healthy weight loss while promoting long-term lifestyle changesA weight loss diet typically focuses on reducing calorie intake while maintaining balanced nutrition to promote fat loss and overall health. Such a diet often includes:

1. Portion control: Paying attention to portion sizes to prevent overeating.

2. Whole foods: Emphasizing fruits, vegetables, lean proteins, and whole grains for their nutrient density and filling properties.

3. Limiting processed foods: Cutting back on sugary snacks, processed meats, and high-calorie, low-nutrient foods.

4. Healthy fats: Incorporating sources of healthy fats like avocados, nuts, seeds, and olive oil for satiety and essential nutrients.

5. Hydration: Drinking plenty of water throughout the day to stay hydrated and support metabolism.

6. Regular meals: Eating balanced meals and snacks at consistent times to maintain energy levels and prevent excessive hunger.

7. Physical activity: Pairing dietary changes with regular exercise to enhance weight loss and overall well-being.

8. Mindful eating: Being aware of hunger and fullness cues, and practicing mindful eating to prevent emotional or mindless eating.

It's important to consult with a healthcare professional or registered dietitian before starting any weight loss diet to ensure it's safe and tailored to individual needs and health goals.

Basic weight loss nutrition

Basic weight loss nutrition focuses on creating a calorie deficit while ensuring adequate intake of essential nutrients. Here are some fundamental principles:

1. Calorie Deficit: To lose weight, you need to consume fewer calories than your body expends. This can be achieved by reducing portion sizes, choosing lower-calorie foods, and increasing physical activity.

2. Balanced Macronutrients: Aim for a balance of carbohydrates, proteins, and fats in your diet. Carbohydrates provide energy, proteins support muscle repair and growth, and fats are essential for hormone production and nutrient absorption.

3. Portion Control: Be mindful of portion sizes to avoid overeating. Use tools like measuring cups, food scales, or hand-size comparisons to gauge appropriate serving sizes.

4. Nutrient-Dense Foods: Focus on foods that provide a high amount of nutrients relative to their calorie content. Examples include fruits, vegetables, lean proteins, whole grains, and healthy fats.

Meal plan

Here's a sample balanced meal plan for weight loss:

Breakfast:

- Scrambled tofu with spinach, tomatoes, and mushrooms
- Whole grain toast
- A small piece of fruit (e.g., apple or berries)
- Green tea or black coffee

Mid-Morning Snack:

- Greek yogurt with a handful of almonds and a drizzle of honey

Lunch:

- Grilled chicken breast
- Quinoa salad with mixed vegetables (bell peppers, cucumber, cherry tomatoes)
- Mixed leafy greens with balsamic vinaigrette dressing

Afternoon Snack:

- Carrot sticks and hummus

Dinner:

- Baked salmon fillet with lemon and herbs
- Steamed broccoli and cauliflower
- Brown rice or sweet potato

Evening Snack (Optional):

- Air-popped popcorn seasoned with a sprinkle of nutritional yeast

Hydration:

- Drink plenty of water throughout the day, aiming for at least 8 glasses.

Notes:

- This meal plan includes a balance of macronutrients (carbohydrates, proteins, fats) to keep you feeling satisfied and energized throughout the day.
- Portion sizes should be adjusted based on individual caloric needs and activity levels.
- Incorporate a variety of fruits, vegetables, lean proteins, and whole grains to ensure you're getting a wide range of nutrients.
- Avoid sugary snacks and beverages, and limit added sugars in your meals.
- Remember to listen to your body's hunger and fullness cues, and adjust your portions accordingly.
- Consult with a healthcare professional or registered dietitian before starting any weight loss meal plan to ensure it's safe and suitable for your individual needs and goals.

Fruit and vegetables for weight loss

Fruits and vegetables are excellent choices for weight loss due to their low calorie density, high fiber content, and abundance of essential vitamins and minerals. Here are some fruits and vegetables particularly beneficial for weight loss:

1. Berries: Berries like strawberries, blueberries, raspberries, and blackberries are low in calories and high in fiber and antioxidants, making them a great choice for satisfying sweet cravings without excess calories.

2. Leafy Greens: Leafy greens such as spinach, kale, Swiss chard, and arugula are nutrient-dense and low in calories. They're rich in vitamins, minerals, and antioxidants, while also providing fiber to promote satiety.

3. Cruciferous Vegetables: Vegetables like broccoli, cauliflower, Brussels sprouts, and cabbage are high in fiber and water content, which can help you feel full while consuming fewer calories. They're also packed with nutrients and offer numerous health benefits.

4. Citrus Fruits: Citrus fruits like oranges, grapefruits, and lemons are low in calories and high in vitamin C and fiber. Their tangy flavor adds brightness to dishes, and their fiber content aids in digestion and promotes feelings of fullness.

5. Apples: Apples are a convenient and satisfying snack option for weight loss. They're high in fiber and water content, which helps you feel full, and they provide natural sweetness without added sugars.

6. Avocado: Although higher in calories than most fruits and vegetables, avocados are rich in healthy fats, fiber, and potassium. Including moderate portions of avocado in your diet can enhance satiety and promote overall health.

7. Bell Peppers: Bell peppers are low in calories and high in fiber and water content. They come in various colors and are packed with vitamins A and C, making them a nutritious addition to salads, stir-fries, and snacks.

Incorporating a variety of fruits and vegetables into your diet can help you feel satisfied while supporting your weight loss goals. Aim to fill half of your plate with fruits and vegetables at each meal to increase volume and nutrient intake while managing calorie consumption.

Foods to limit and avoid

When aiming for weight loss, it's important to limit or avoid certain foods that are high in calories, sugar, unhealthy fats, and processed ingredients. Here are some foods to limit or avoid:

1. Processed Foods: Processed foods like chips, cookies, cakes, and pastries are often high in calories, sugar, unhealthy fats, and additives. They provide little nutritional value and can lead to weight gain when consumed in excess.

2. Sugar-Sweetened Beverages: Sugary drinks such as soda, fruit juices, energy drinks, and sweetened teas are loaded with added sugars and calories. These beverages contribute to weight gain and are linked to an increased risk of obesity, type 2 diabetes, and other health issues.

3. Fast Food and Fried Foods: Fast food meals and fried foods like burgers, fries, fried chicken, and pizza are typically high in calories, unhealthy fats, and sodium. Consuming these foods frequently can lead to weight gain and negative health outcomes.

4. White Bread and Refined Grains: White bread, white rice, pasta, and other refined grains have been stripped of their fiber and nutrients during processing, leaving behind simple carbohydrates that can spike blood sugar levels and promote weight gain. Opt for whole grains instead, which are higher in fiber and nutrients.

5. Processed Meats: Processed meats such as bacon, sausage, hot dogs, deli meats, and certain packaged meats contain high levels of sodium, saturated fats, and preservatives. These meats have been linked to an increased risk of heart disease, cancer, and weight gain.

6. Sauces, Condiments, and Dressings: Many sauces, condiments, and salad dressings are high in calories, sugar, and unhealthy fats. Be mindful of portion sizes and choose options with minimal added sugars and unhealthy fats.

7. High-Calorie Snacks: Snack foods like potato chips, candy bars, chocolate, and ice cream are high in calories, sugar, and unhealthy fats. Opt for healthier snack options such as nuts, seeds, fruits, vegetables, and yogurt.

By limiting or avoiding these foods and focusing on whole, nutrient-dense options, you can support your weight loss efforts and improve your overall health and well-being. Remember to read food labels and choose foods that are lower in added sugars, unhealthy fats, and processed ingredients.

Beverages and weight loss

Choosing the right beverages can support your weight loss efforts by helping you stay hydrated, controlling your appetite, and providing essential nutrients without excess calories. Here are some beverages that can aid in weight loss:

1. Water: Water is essential for hydration and can help boost metabolism, suppress appetite, and promote feelings of fullness. Drinking water before meals may also help reduce calorie intake.
2. Green Tea: Green tea is rich in antioxidants called catechins, which have been shown to promote fat burning and increase metabolism. Drinking green tea regularly may aid in weight loss and improve overall health.
3. Black Coffee: Coffee is low in calories and can temporarily boost metabolism, leading to increased calorie burning. However, be

mindful of added sugars and high-calorie creamers. Opt for black coffee or add a splash of unsweetened almond milk for flavor.

4. Herbal Tea: Herbal teas like peppermint, chamomile, and ginger tea are calorie-free and can help promote relaxation, reduce stress, and support digestion, all of which may contribute to weight loss.

5. Vegetable Juice: Freshly squeezed vegetable juices, such as carrot, celery, and kale juice, can provide essential nutrients and hydration without excess calories. Just be mindful of portion sizes and avoid adding extra sugar or sweeteners.

6. Protein Shakes: Protein shakes made with protein powder, water or unsweetened almond milk, and added fruits or vegetables can be a convenient and filling option for weight loss. Protein helps keep you feeling full and satisfied, which can prevent overeating.

7. Sparkling Water: Sparkling water or seltzer can be a refreshing alternative to sugary sodas and juices. Look for unsweetened varieties and add a splash of lemon or lime juice for flavor.

8. Coconut Water: Coconut water is low in calories and rich in electrolytes, making it a hydrating beverage option. However, it's important to choose unsweetened varieties to avoid added sugars.

When selecting beverages for weight loss, it's essential to prioritize hydration and choose options that are low in calories and added sugars. Be mindful of portion sizes and avoid excessive consumption of high-calorie beverages like sugary sodas, energy drinks, and alcoholic beverages.

Exercises

Incorporating regular exercise into your routine is essential for weight loss, as it helps increase calorie expenditure, improve metabolism, and preserve lean muscle mass. Here are some effective exercises for weight loss:

1. Cardiovascular Exercise: Cardio workouts are great for burning calories and improving cardiovascular health. Examples include:
   - Brisk walking or jogging
   - Cycling
   - I'm Swimming
   - Running
   - Jumping rope
   - Dancing
   - Aerobic classes

2. High-Intensity Interval Training (HIIT): HIIT involves alternating between short bursts of intense exercise and periods of rest or lower-intensity activity. This type of workout can help burn more calories in less time and boost metabolism. Examples include:
   - HIIT circuits (e.g., burpees, jumping jacks, mountain climbers)
   - Sprint intervals (e.g., running or cycling sprints followed by recovery periods)
   - Tabata workouts (e.g., 20 seconds of high-intensity exercise followed by 10 seconds of rest, repeated for multiple rounds)
3. Strength Training: Building lean muscle mass through strength training helps increase metabolism and promote fat loss. Incorporate exercises that target major muscle groups, such as:
   - Squats
   - Lunges
   - Deadlifts
   - Bench presses
   - Rows
   - Pull-ups/chin-ups
   - Push-ups
   - Planks

4. Bodyweight Exercises: Bodyweight exercises are effective for strength training and can be done anywhere with minimal equipment. Examples include:

   - Bodyweight squats
   - Push-ups
   - Lunges
   - Planks
   - Glute bridges
   - Tricep dips
   - Mountain climbers

5. Flexibility and Mobility Exercises: Stretching and mobility exercises can help improve flexibility, reduce muscle tension, and prevent injuries. Incorporate activities like yoga, Pilates, or dynamic stretching into your routine to enhance overall fitness and recovery.

6. Active Lifestyle: In addition to structured exercise sessions, focus on increasing daily physical activity by incorporating more movement into your routine. Take the stairs instead of the elevator, walk or bike instead of driving short distances, and find ways to stay active throughout the day.

Remember to consult with a healthcare professional before starting any new exercise program, especially if you have any underlying health conditions or concerns. Aim for a balanced approach that includes a mix of cardiovascular exercise, strength training, flexibility work, and daily movement to support your weight loss goals and overall health.

Overcoming challenges and plateaus

Overcoming challenges and plateaus in weight loss requires persistence, patience, and a willingness to adapt. Here are some strategies to help you push through obstacles and continue making progress:

1. Evaluate Your Habits: Take a step back and assess your current habits, including dietary choices, exercise routines, stress levels, and sleep patterns. Identify any areas where you may be struggling or could make improvements.
2. Set Realistic Goals: Adjust your weight loss goals if necessary to make them more achievable and sustainable. Focus on making

gradual progress over time rather than aiming for rapid weight loss, which can be difficult to maintain.

3. Diversify Your Workouts: Shake up your exercise routine by trying new activities or challenging yourself with different types of workouts. Incorporating variety into your fitness regimen can prevent boredom, stimulate muscle growth, and overcome plateaus.

4. Monitor Your Progress: Keep track of your food intake, exercise habits, and weight loss progress to identify patterns and make adjustments as needed. Use a journal, app, or wearable fitness tracker to monitor your daily habits and stay accountable.

5. Focus on Non-Scale Victories: Instead of solely focusing on the number on the scale, celebrate other indicators of progress such as improved energy levels, increased strength and endurance, better sleep, and enhanced mood.

6. Manage Stress: Stress can negatively impact weight loss efforts by increasing cortisol levels and triggering emotional eating. Practice stress-reduction techniques such as meditation, deep breathing exercises, yoga, or spending time in nature to promote relaxation and improve overall well-being.

7. Get Adequate Sleep: Prioritize quality sleep, as inadequate sleep can disrupt hunger hormones, increase cravings for unhealthy foods, and hinder weight loss efforts. Aim for 7-9 hours of sleep per night and establish a consistent sleep schedule.

8. Stay Hydrated: Drink plenty of water throughout the day to stay hydrated and support metabolism. Sometimes thirst can be mistaken for hunger, so staying hydrated can help prevent overeating.

9. Seek Support: Surround yourself with a supportive network of friends, family, or a weight loss support group who can provide encouragement, accountability, and motivation during challenging times.

10. Be Patient and Persistent: Remember that weight loss is not always linear, and progress may occur gradually over time. Stay committed to your goals, stay positive, and trust in the process.

By implementing these strategies and staying focused on your long-term goals, you can overcome challenges and plateaus in weight loss and continue moving forward on your journey to better health.

Conclusion

In conclusion, embarking on a weight loss diet represents far more than just a numerical goal of shedding excess pounds. It embodies a profound commitment to transforming one's relationship with food, lifestyle, and ultimately, their own well-being. The journey towards sustainable weight loss is multifaceted, requiring a holistic approach that encompasses nutrition, physical activity, mindset, and self-care.

First and foremost, a weight loss diet is about nourishing the body with nutrient-dense foods that fuel energy, support metabolism, and promote overall health. It involves making conscious choices to prioritize whole, unprocessed foods rich in vitamins, minerals, fiber, and essential nutrients, while minimizing intake of empty calories, refined sugars, and unhealthy fats. By embracing a diet abundant in fruits, vegetables, lean proteins, whole grains, and healthy fats, individuals lay the foundation for sustainable weight loss and long-term health.

Moreover, portion control and mindful eating are fundamental aspects of a successful weight loss journey. Learning to listen to hunger and satiety cues, practicing mindful eating techniques, and being aware of emotional triggers can help prevent overeating and promote a healthier relationship with food. By savoring each bite, enjoying meals without distractions, and honoring the body's signals of hunger and fullness, individuals cultivate a deeper connection to their dietary choices and enhance their ability to make informed decisions that support their weight loss goals.

In addition to dietary changes, regular physical activity plays a crucial role in achieving and maintaining weight loss. Exercise not only helps burn calories and promote fat loss but also strengthens muscles, improves cardiovascular health, boosts mood, and enhances overall well-being. Incorporating a variety of cardiovascular, strength training, and flexibility exercises into one's routine can maximize calorie expenditure, stimulate metabolism, and contribute to long-term weight management.

Furthermore, navigating the challenges and plateaus inherent in the weight loss journey requires resilience, patience, and self-compassion. It's essential to recognize that setbacks are a natural part of the process and to approach them with a growth mindset, viewing them as opportunities for learning and growth rather than reasons for discouragement. By staying focused on long-term goals, celebrating non-scale victories, and seeking support from friends, family, or professional resources when needed, individuals can overcome obstacles and continue progressing towards their desired outcomes.

Ultimately, a weight loss diet is not a one-size-fits-all approach but rather a deeply personal journey that requires individualized strategies and a commitment to self-care. It's about empowering oneself to make healthier choices, cultivate sustainable habits, and embrace a lifestyle that prioritizes both physical and emotional well-being. By embracing the principles of balanced nutrition, mindful eating, regular exercise, and self-compassion, individuals can embark on a transformative journey towards lasting weight loss success and a brighter, healthier future.

FAQ

Certainly! Here are some frequently asked questions (FAQs) on weight loss diet:

1. What is a weight loss diet?
   - A weight loss diet is a structured eating plan designed to help individuals lose weight by reducing calorie intake while maintaining balanced nutrition.
2. How does a weight loss diet work?
   - A weight loss diet works by creating a calorie deficit, where you consume fewer calories than your body needs for maintenance, prompting it to burn stored fat for energy.
3. What foods should I eat on a weight loss diet?

- Focus on whole, nutrient-dense foods such as fruits, vegetables, lean proteins, whole grains, and healthy fats. These foods provide essential nutrients while keeping you feeling full and satisfied.

4. How much weight can I expect to lose on a weight loss diet?

    - Weight loss varies depending on factors such as starting weight, metabolic rate, activity level, and adherence to the diet plan. A safe and sustainable rate of weight loss is typically 1-2 pounds per week.

5. Are there specific foods I should avoid on a weight loss diet?

    - Limit or avoid foods high in added sugars, unhealthy fats, and processed ingredients, such as sugary snacks, fried foods, white bread, and sugary beverages.

6. Do I need to count calories on a weight loss diet?

    - While calorie counting can be a helpful tool for some individuals, it's not always necessary. Focus on portion control, mindful eating, and choosing nutrient-dense foods to support weight loss.

7. How important is exercise for weight loss?

- Exercise plays a crucial role in weight loss by increasing calorie expenditure, boosting metabolism, and preserving lean muscle mass. Aim for a combination of cardiovascular exercise, strength training, and flexibility work for optimal results.

8. How can I stay motivated on a weight loss diet?

- Set realistic goals, track your progress, celebrate milestones, find support from friends or online communities, and focus on non-scale victories such as improved energy levels and mood.

9. What should I do if I hit a weight loss plateau?

- If you hit a plateau, reassess your habits, adjust your diet and exercise routine as needed, and consider consulting with a healthcare professional or registered dietitian for personalized guidance.

10. Is it possible to maintain weight loss long-term?

- Yes, maintaining weight loss long-term is possible by adopting sustainable lifestyle habits, such as regular exercise, balanced nutrition, portion control, and mindful eating.

These are just a few common questions related to weight loss diets, and seeking guidance from healthcare professionals or registered dietitians can provide personalized advice and support.